A Guide To Giving Up Smoking

A Guide To Giving Up Smoking

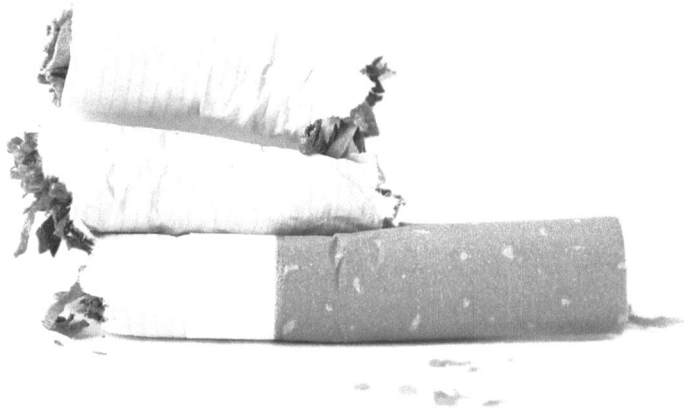

JAMES DOWNIE

A Guide To Giving Up Smoking

ISBN: 978-1-922159-19-9

See other books by the Author at his Amazon author page:
www.amazon.com/author/bestselling

Published by Blue Peg Publishing

If you have purchased the ebook version of this book, then please consider buying the print version if your family enjoys the ebook.

Contents

CHAPTER ONE

Answer This: Why Do You Want To Quit?

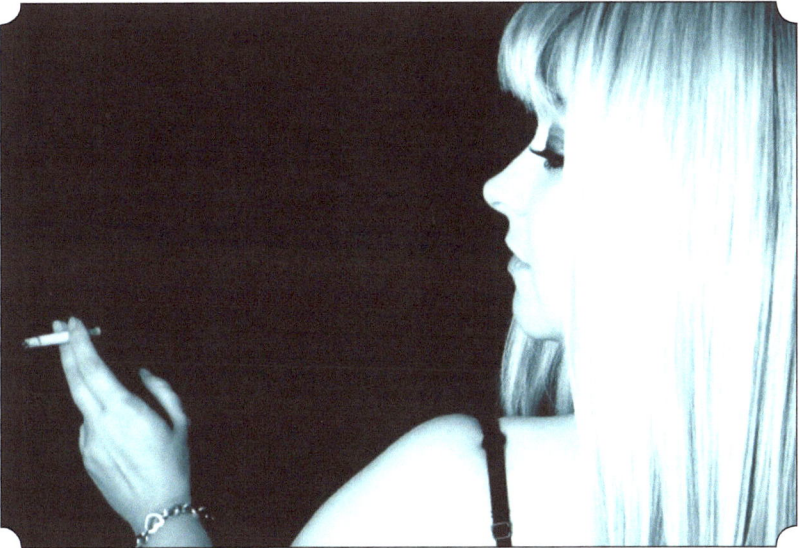

Everyone assumes you want to quit smoking because it is bad for your health.

That's not how it happens.

If you are the kind of person who is really fearful about your health, you would never have started. Or, if you were lured into smoking as a youngster by your peers, you would have stopped as soon as you read a single warning from the World Health Organization or the Surgeon General of your country.

The reality is that your reason for deciding to quit at this precise time of your life is as individual as you are.

You may have fallen in love with someone with asthma who can't bear to be close to you because even the smell on your clothes prompts an attack.

Your three-year-old may have said "Yukky Daddy, you stink" when you stepped back into the house after a smoke, and you decided then and there to change.

Your spouse may be suffering from the effects of your second hand smoke. Your sister may have been diagnosed with lung cancer. Your best buddy may have just died from cancer caused by smoking.

You may want to take a 14-hour flight to see a country you have always dreamed of visiting, but you know you can't smoke on the flight and you can't go that long without a cigarette.

You may have just done the math and realized in the last 10 years you spent close to $40,000 on cigarettes and realized that your house would be paid off now had you quit earlier.

Basically, you quit smoking for all the big reasons you do anything in life: love, money, sex, and a shot at living longer and having more fun. It's not complicated.

Regardless of what prompted you at this point and time in your life to quit, this book can help you. We have researched all the latest studies and publications on quitting techniques and assembled them in an easy-to-read, straightforward guide to help you give up smoking.

As you work your way through the chapters, you will learn to understand what smoking has done to your body, and what you can expect in the days and weeks that follow your last cigarette, cigar or pipe of tobacco.

You will learn techniques to help you cope with the cravings and the social stresses that follow such a significant lifestyle change as quitting smoking.

Most importantly, we will help you devise your own quitting plan and prepare strategies tailor made to your personality.

We will look at ways to avoid the stress and depression that follow withdrawal from smoking, and ways to manage your weight so that you do not substitute your craving for cigarettes with a craving for food.

If you are just thinking about quitting, but haven't yet set the date, this is a great way to get a grasp on what you can expect and how to handle the challenges that go with quitting.

If you have just stopped smoking, this book will help you formulate strategies for the tough weeks ahead.

If you quit a few months but fight relapsing every day, we will offer strategies for your long-term success.

At the foundation of our guide to giving up smoking is a recognition of the importance of figuring out your unique, personal reason for quitting. This matters greatly because you will need tremendous motivation to succeed, and this reason will ultimately be the source of your deepest and most persistent motivation.

So take some time at the beginning and figure out your personal reason for quitting. Be honest with yourself. This is not a reason you have to share with other people unless you want to; it is your own private source of strength for the weeks to come.

If you need other reasons, there are lots of them. Start with the stark reality that somebody dies from tobacco use every eight seconds, according to the <u>World Health Organization</u>. It shouldn't be you.

Around the globe, smoking-related diseases kill one out of every 10 adults, or four million people a year. If the current trend continues, smoking will be killing one out of every six people in the near future.

Despite these sobering realities, about a third of the male adult global population smokes. About 15 billion cigarettes are sold every day, or 10 million each minute.

Smoking is increasing in the developing world, but declining in developed nations like United States, Britain, Australia and Canada. The highest smoking rate now is in the Western Pacific Region.

Every cigarette you smoke cuts at least five minutes off your life, on average. That's about the time it takes to smoke it.

You know it's time to stop. You know why you really want to stop.

You will be even more firm in your resolve if you round off your personal reasons with other concerns based on scientific studies. In the quitting business, it's called building a foundation case.

- You need facts to support your case:

Smoking does a lot of bad things to your health. Many of them are outlined in a report called "The Health Consequences of Smoking: A Report of the U.S. Surgeon General."

If you quit, here are some of the things you can accomplish for yourself:

- Reduce your risk of having a stroke: Smokers are four times more likely than non-smokers to have a stroke. Non-smokers living with smokers are also more likely to have a stroke. Strokes are horrible things. They make part of your brain die and it often doesn't come back. You might have paralysis of parts of your body or be unable to speak clearly. You can also die of a stroke. Between five and 15 years after quitting smoking, your risk of having a stroke is the same as a non-smoker.

- Heighten your chances of not going blind: If you smoke, you are four times more likely to develop age-related macular degeneration. It is a disease that affects the macular, the central part of the retina at the back of the eye that gives you the vision for such tasks as driving, reading and recognizing faces. When it happens, it stays that way. There is no cure. The number of years you smoke and the number of cigarettes you smoke increases your risk. Smoking also increases your risk of developing cataracts, a leading cause of blindness.

- Lower your odds of getting mouth and throat cancers: More than 80 percent of cancers of the mouth, nose, and throat occur in people who smoke cigarettes, cigars and pipes. Smokers are also at greater risk of developing cancer of the esophagus, larynx (voice box,) tongue, lips and salivary glands. If you smoke, you are nine times more likely to develop one of these cancers. If you smoke a pack a day, you are 16 times more apt to get cancer of the larynx. Smoking also causes gum disease and bad breath.

- Avoid dying a horrible death from lung cancer: Most lung cancers are caused by smoking, and most of them are fatal. The younger you were when you started smoking, the more likely you are to develop lung cancer. Your risk of developing lung cancer drops by up to 50 percent within 10 years of when you quit smoking. Your second-hand smoke also causes lung cancer in the non-smokers who live and work with you. Smoking also causes other serious lung diseases like chronic bronchitis and emphysema.

- Lower the likelihood of having a heart attack: Smoking leads to the development of atherosclerosis, the narrowing and clogging of your arteries, and this causes heart disease and strokes. People who smoke are 150 percent more likely to develop heart disease than those who don't. Smokers have more heart attacks, repeat heart attacks and more than 20 times the angina than non-smokers. Smokers have heart attacks at a much younger age than non-smokers. Smokers are four times more likely to die of coronary heart disease than non-smokers. Even smoking one cigarette increases your heart rate, prompts a short-term increase in your blood pressure, and decreases the oxygen in your blood.

After one year of quitting smoking, your risk of heart disease is halved. Fifteen years after you quit, your risk is the same as a non-smoker.

- Increase your chances of having a healthy baby: Men who smoke are more likely to develop impotence (erectile dysfunction) than non-smokers because of the reduced blood flow to the penis caused by atherosclerosis. As well, 30 percent of penile cancer in men is estimated to be attributed to smoking. Recent students also suggest that smoking may affect the development and quality of sperm, decrease the sperm count, and reduce the volume of semen. Toxins found in tobacco smoke such as cadmium, nicotine, benzopyrene and their by-products can damage the genetic material in sperm cells. Students also suggest that children of fathers who smoke have a greater chance of developing childhood cancers.

For women, smoking during pregnancy reduces the growth and health of babies and increases the risk of a number of complications and illnesses for both the mother and baby. Studies show mothers who smoke are twice as likely to have babies with a below-normal birth weight, a leading cause of infant death and a risk factor in other health problems in infancy and childhood. Mothers who smoke are 50 percent more apt to have a stillborn baby compared to mothers who do not. Babies of mothers who smoke before and after birth are three times more likely to die from Sudden Infant Death Syndrome. As well, smoking causes problems for women's reproductive systems including difficulty conceiving, earlier menopause and increased risk of cervical and vulval cancer. Smoking has also been linked to menstrual cycle irregularities.

It's easy to augment your case. Whatever your primary motivation for quitting is, you can add a host of other reasons from the above list to firm up your resolve. Any one of them can stand on its own, but taken together, they build the foundation for your personal plan to giving up smoking.

Keep in mind as well that unlike many other lifestyle changes that take ages to have an impact on your life, when you quit smoking, good things happen in your body right away.

Here is a quick list of improvements that you will start to enjoy within hours of smoking your last cigarette.

Ten Ways Your Body Benefits As Soon As You Quit Smoking

1. Almost all of the harmful nicotine will be out of your system within 12 hours.

2. You will have more oxygen in your bloodstream within 24 hours and the level of carbon monoxide in your blood will drop dramatically.

3. Most of the harmful nicotine by-products will be gone from your body within five days.

4. Your sense of taste and smell improves in less than one week.

5. Your blood pressure will return to its normal level within one month.

6. Your immune system will start to show vital signs of recovery within one month.

7. Your lungs will no longer be producing extra phlegm caused by smoking within two months after quitting.

8. Your risk of dying from heart disease will be half that of a continuing smoke after 12 months of not smoking.

9. Your risk of lung cancer will be less than half that of a continuing smoker within 10 years of quitting and it will continue to decline after 10 years of quitting.

10. Your risk of heart attack and stroke will be almost the same as that of a person who has never smoked within 15 years of quitting.

CHAPTER TWO

Do Some Sleuthing On Your Current Smoking Habit

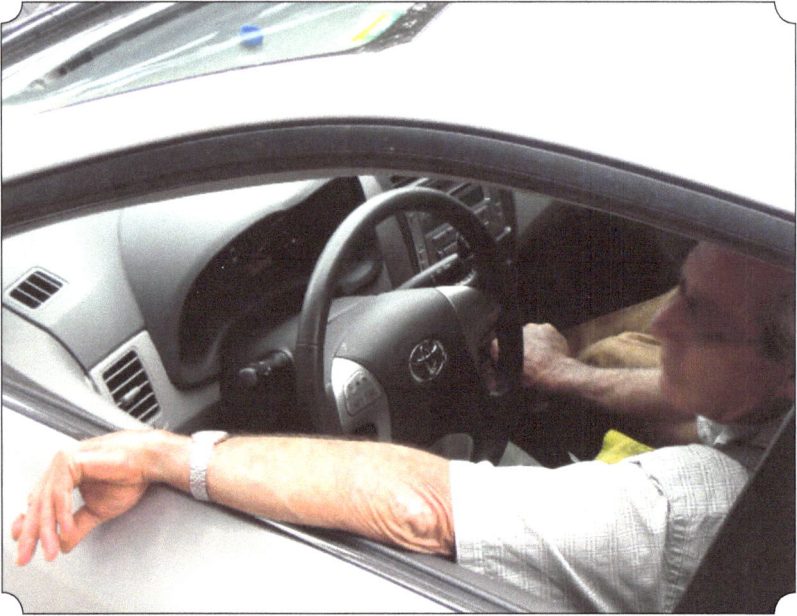

In the early morning air, have you ever blown a smoke ring and idly watched as it curled its way around a myriad of objects in its path? You wonder how something as fragile as a whiff of smoke could touch so many things and go so far on a current of air.

When you smoke, your habit is a bit like that smoke ring. It touches so many parts of your life, weaving and interweaving with who you are, what you do, and who you do it with.

You may think that you smoke alone. You may think that it is an individual choice and your decision to smoke is yours and yours alone. You may re-enforce this when you smoke alone in the privacy of your living room or at a sidewalk cafe with your favourite cup of coffee.

So you think that quitting will be a personal, private project. But it rarely works out that way.

That is because smoking touches many more parts of your life than you realize. When you decide to quit, it impacts the heart and soul of you, the people you live with, the people you play with, and the people you work with.

It impacts parts of your body that act as if you no longer have any control of them. It impacts your emotions and your deepest sense of self. It impacts your comfort zone, and if you have taken no thought on how to find a new one, it will tear away at you, often creating depression or a substitute addiction for food or drink.

You may think that you smoke because you have an addiction to nicotine. If you can overcome that, you will succeed.

Sadly, that is not always the case. The loss of a comforting habit, when it is not replaced with another, can lead to depression, a substitute addiction, and ultimately, a return to smoking.

That is why is it vital to do some detective work on your current smoking habit before you quit. Understanding what makes you smoke (over and above the nicotine craving), will allow you to build a more solid plan of action and greatly increase your chances of success.

Most people have four triggers that make them reach for a cigarette, cigar or pipe.

The strongest of these is their emotions. Feeling stressed? Have a cigarette and the very process of inhaling and exhaling will calm you. Are you upset? Same thing. If you are frustrated, picking yourself up and going outside for a change of scenery and a cigarette can help you see the problem with new, calmer and more creative eyes when you return.

How many times, in real life and in movies, have you seen a leading man being visibly bored at a social function move out to a patio and light up a cigarette, a welcome "time out" from a scene they no longer want to be in? Do you smoke at the end of the day when you are sitting in your car in a traffic jam, bored and tired and just wanting to be home?

On the opposite side of the specter, are you more inclined to smoke when you are happy? Is it your little way of celebrating a report finished, a job well done, a great meal eaten, or a challenge completed?

All of our emotions, from sadness to happiness, from boredom to anxiety, from frustration to celebration, can be triggers for reaching for a cigarette.

Pleasure is another major trigger for smokers. In the glow of great sex, do you light up a cigarette to savour the feeling of the moment? On the city apartment balcony or on your rural front porch, do you love to light up and have a peaceful smoke as you watch the sunset, contemplating the end of a great day?

The third and fourth most common triggers to smokers are social pressure and habit.

Now that so many workplaces have banned smoking, a counter culture has sprung up involving the smokers who meet outside two or three times a day to share their lives and cigarettes. Are you part of a good little group of friends who break up your work day with these smoke breaks? Will your friendships all change if you no longer smoke?

When you and your friends get together for drinks at a neighbourhood bar, are all of you smoking? When you go on a "girl's night out" or to a card party, are cigarettes and beer the standard fare? How will you feel having one without the other? Can you cope with the smell and sight of them enjoying cigarettes when you are not? Will you still feel comfortable participating in these rituals of your life?

Many smokers also have a habit of having a cigarette when they are doing certain routine things in their lives. For example, do you love to have a cigarette when you are puttering in your workshop? Do you reward yourself when the kids have left for school every morning with a cup of great coffee and a cigarette?

As a general rule, it takes about two weeks for most people to get a realistic handle on when they smoke, how much they smoke, and what triggers their need to smoke.

Invest in a small notebook and sleuth on your smoking habits for a couple of weeks. Keep a record of when you have a cigarette, and the circumstances of where and when you smoked. With each entry, write down one of the four triggers (emotions, pleasure, social pressure and habit) that comes closest to describing the category this smoking session fell into.

Leave a few lines after each entry. At whatever point of the day you have a little quiet time, look at the entries and ask yourself two questions:

1. If I hadn't smoked at that time, would that emotional trigger have been satisfied?
2. If I hadn't smoked at that time, would I have enjoyed that situation as much?

It is vitally important to understand your smoking habits so you will be better prepared to handle the trigger points when you quit. Knowing what it is that makes you want to smoke will help you better figure out a strategy to cope with these same situations when you don't want to smoke.

If it is easier for you to keep an online diary, Quit Victoria, an initiative of the Australian Department of Human Services, the Cancer Council Victoria, the National Heart Foundation and the Victoria Health Promotion Foundation offers a workable, downloadable Smoker Diary.

They suggest that besides recording the date and time of each cigarette and the activity or situation you are in when you smoke, you also record what you are feeling and how much you feel the need for that cigarette, on a scale of one to five, with five being the most needed.

While it is recommended you keep this diary for two weeks, you will have a good idea of what makes you want to smoke and how badly within a couple of days.

This information is vital to your quitting plan. It is you record of your personalized smoking triggers. By looking over this information, it will be very clear to you which times and which situations will be the toughest for you once you quit.

When you sit down to complete your individual quitting plan, one of the things you will have to consider is how you will cope with those specific situations. You need to think of a plan in advance to deal with your trigger situations.

While you are doing your detective work on your current smoking habit, think about one other detail of your habit. What does your smoking cost you in a day, a week, a month, a year?

If you put that money in a savings bank each month, what would you like to use it for at the end of the first or second year? Would you plan a trip, buy a car, remodel your home? What big goal would be appealing to you?

Many quitters get through their toughest days by focusing on something as concrete as a financial reward. While it is appealing to know that you are reducing your risk of having a heart attack, somehow it doesn't spark the same emotional response as knowing you can take the kids to Disney World after one year if you can just stick to your goal.

CHAPTER THREE

Decide How You Will Deal With Your Nicotine Addiction

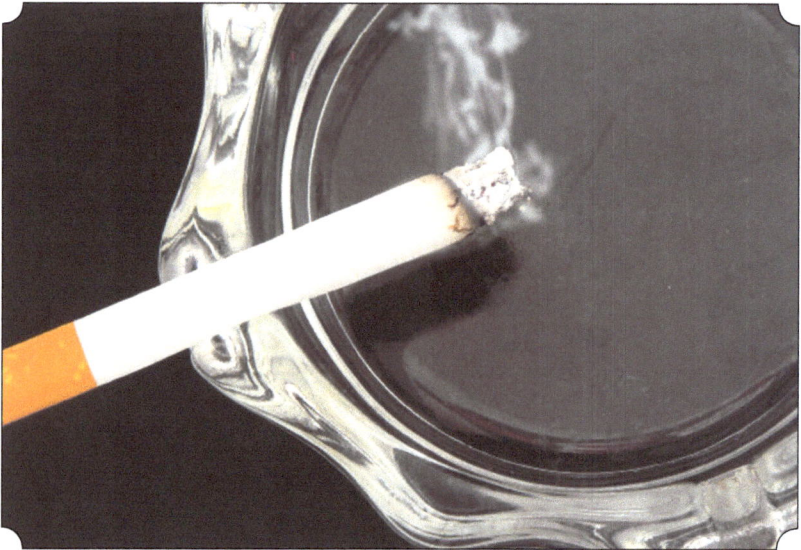

If you have decided to quit smoking, you likely believe that whether you succeed or fail will ultimately come down to your strength or weakness.

In reality, it's not about that at all.

It's about how you handle your dopamine pathway receptors' attraction to nicotine molecules.

That doesn't sound as heroic or even as straightforward, but it is the key to the science of quitting.

When you decide to quit smoking, the most important thing you have to simultaneously consider is how you will deal with your nicotine addiction. There are forces within you as a smoker stronger than you realize, fuelled by a powerful drug that has control of your brain.

It is a good idea to take some time in the planning stages to learn about nicotine and what it does to your body and your brain, and then look at strategies for wrestling control from it.

Nicotine is the addictive substance in cigarette smoke that makes you its slave. It is present in the tobacco leaf itself and is in fact the plant's protection from insects. Used as a natural insecticide by farmers, it is now being blamed for the death of honey bees in great numbers. When you burn tobacco, the nicotine enters your body through the smoke you inhale.

It moves fast. Within 10 seconds after you inhale it, it has entered your bloodstream by way of your lungs and made its way directly to your brain. There it sets to work changing the structure and function of your brain. In a flash, it assumes control of the flow of more than 200 neuro-chemicals, including dopamine.

It then makes you feel good and then it makes you feel bad, and it does that perversely in a cycle that swings you from cigarette to cigarette, hour to hour, day to day, week to week. It enslaves you in its cycle of power.

When you first smoke that cigarette, you revel in its positive power. You feel relaxed, more focused and perhaps even aroused. But after awhile you notice its negative forces. You feel irritable, nervous, restless, anxious and unfocused.

17

Its control begins immediately and its hold is fast. In fact, nicotine is more than likely to make you an addict than your first dose of cocaine, beer, or marijuana.

The younger you start smoking, the more powerfully nicotine exerts its strength and power in your body and brain. Studies show teen smokers are especially vulnerable to the effects of this substance.

The thrill you experience when the nicotine hits your brain wears off quickly because the substance moves through the rest of your body and is metabolised. When that happens, you feel nicotine withdrawal. You smoke another cigarette to relieve the withdrawal symptoms, and you feel great for a short period of time, but then the cycle starts again.

If you smoke a pack or more a day, this cycle of feeling great followed by withdrawal marks your day more than a hundred times. It is no wonder that so many people end up smoking themselves to death rather than deal with the hell that is breaking the cycle.

If you switched to a low nicotine/tar cigarette brand, you haven't solved anything. What happens in this instance is that you still seek for the fulfilling nicotine level, because your brain and body wants it, so you inhale even more cigarette smoke and you inhale deeper.

Besides the perils of nicotine, you also have to rid your body of the other cancer-causing substances you inhale each time you smoke.

Tobacco smoke contains more than 4,000 chemicals and more than 60 of them have been directly identified as causing cancer in animals. Eleven of them have been positively identified as cancer-causing in humans, and another eight are suspected of causing cancer in humans.

Just as the nicotine makes its way all through your body, so do the toxins in the cigarette smoke itself. They go everywhere your blood goes. They make you sick by interrupting normal cell growth, the precursor of cancer cells forming.

According to the <u>American Council on Science and Health</u>, the chemicals you inhale that will make you ill are benzene, 2-naphthylamine, 4-aminobiphenyl, chromium, cadmium, vinyl chloride, ethylene oxide, arsenic, beryllium, nickel and polonium-210.12.

Other parts of the chemical stew you breath in with every cigarette, besides the nicotine, include formaldehyde, used to preserve dead laboratory specimens, ammonia, used in toilet cleaners, hydrogen cyanide, used in rat poison, acetone, used in nail polish remover, carbon monoxide, found in car exhaust, tar, used to pave roads, toluene, used in paint thinners and phenol, used in fertilizers. None of these are good for you.

Smoking pipes or cigars doesn't let you off the hook either. Smoking tobacco in any form still causes cancer. Any differences in statistics have been identified as related to differences in daily use and level of inhalation. Remember that the composition of smoke analyzed from cigars and cigarettes is essentially the same. Smoking five cigars a day is the equivalent to smoking a pack of cigarettes in terms of the number of toxins entering your body.

The ingestion of smoke into your bloodstream also damages the blood vessels in your body. This damage to the blood vessels that supply the arms and legs leads to an illness called <u>Peripheral Vascular Disease</u> (PVD) and it occurs most often in the legs and feet.

It causes severe pain and as it progresses, it can cause sores in the legs and feet not to heal and gangrene can set in. Amputation is the next step.

So you want to quit smoking, but the more you learn it is reasonable to wonder if you can possibly succeed against such a powerful protagonist as nicotine. It has you firmly in its grasp, and it is not going to let you slide away so easily.

According to statistics from the World Health Organization, only seven percent of those who quit without support are still smoke free at the end of the first year.

Even among those who succeed, there is never complete independence. Most smokers who slip back and try to have just the occasional cigarette are quickly back to their own routine of smoking a pack or two a day. Like alcoholism or drug addiction, quitting smoking means you can't go back, not even for a little while.

As officials at Australia's <u>QuitNow</u> program put it, there is just one concept, and just one rule.

The concept is that "one is too many and a thousand is never enough."

The rule is simply "no nicotine for just one hour," and it extends day after day, week after week.

You have the will to quit. You know the concept of quitting. You know the rule of quitting. But what else can you know that will ease the days ahead?

You need to know that at the essence of the whole quitting exercises, you have two key problems to overcome:

-   Nicotine dependence and
-   Nicotine withdrawal

Understand that you are currently dependent on nicotine. As soon as you stop inhaling it, you need to find a way to deal with withdrawal. You will feel the symptoms of withdrawal swift and fast. You are going to feel anxious, hungry, and irritable. You may find it very hard to focus on your work or even your life. You may have headaches and have difficulty sleeping. Some people experience a decreased heart rate and blood pressure.

You may also find that you are tired and coughing. Many smokers who just quit wonder why they felt so much better when they were still smoking. What is happening with the coughing and the fatigue is that your body is cleaning out the poisons linked to smoking and repairing itself.

You may want to ease your nicotine withdrawal with such aids as nicotine patches, gums or inhalers, or even prescription medicine. Whether or not it is good to use them is a subject of considerable controversy among health professionals. Many authorities acknowledge that although they ease symptoms, in the end, the smoker still has to get the nicotine out of his system.

You may feel you must try some of them. The important thing is not to become so dependent on them that you drag out the withdrawal period for weeks or months, slowly lowering the nicotine in your system.

The roughest, most severe withdrawal symptoms will take place in the first week after quitting, even though the craving for a cigarette goes on for a much longer time.

These medications won't magically stop all your withdrawal symptoms, but they will ease some of them, especially the cravings, irritability, mood swings and anxiety. And with each passing day, you will grow stronger.

Here is a quick guide to the most common nicotine withdrawal aids:

Nicotine Replacement Therapy – This involves gums, patches, lozenges, and inhalers. The idea is that the person quitting smoking gets low doses of nicotine to stave off the withdrawal symptoms while the body rids itself first of the toxins found in cigarette smoke. Nicotine replacement will ease the cravings along with the symptoms. Scientific studies show that as a general rule, nicotine replacement therapy works best for moderate to heavy smokers who smoked more than 15 cigarettes a day.

The positives are that you are less inclined to cheat the first day you quit smoking, and this alone will increase your chance of stopping for good by tenfold. It also helps prevent weight gain while it is being used, but you are still at risk of weight gain when you stop using all nicotine.

The negatives are that the more cigarettes you smoke, the more of a dose of nicotine replacement you will need at the start of your therapy. You might smoke while using the nicotine replacement patch and this could cause nicotine to build up to toxic levels in your body.

If you decide to use Nicotine Replacement Therapy, remember that the dose of nicotine should be slowly reduced.

Studies also show that people are most likely to use gum and patches correctly.

If you use the patch, replace it every 24 hours at the start. If you smoke less than 10 cigarettes a day, use a lower dose patch to start with. Put the patch on different areas of your body above your waist and below your neck. It takes about two to four hours for the patch to work.

If you use the gum, chew one to two pieces each hour, and no more than 20 pieces a day. Chew the gum slowly until it develops a peppery taste. Then tuck it between you gum and cheek and store it there so the nicotine can be absorb. You should stop using the gum by six months. There is yet no research to confirm that using gum over a long period of time is any safer than smoking. Wait at least 15 minutes after having tea, coffee, colas or acidic beverages before chewing gum.

The nicotine inhaler can be picked up at the counter in many pharmacies around the world, but is available only by prescription in the United States. You insert nicotine cartridges into the inhaler and puff them about 20 minutes up to 16 times a day. The inhaler works faster than the patch. The inhaler causes some people to experience coughing and sore throats. The inhaler and patch can be combined effectively for some people.

The nasal spray can also be used in combination with the patch. Levels of nicotine peak within five to 10 minutes of using it. It can irritate the eyes, nose and throat, but this passes after a few days.

Side effects of all of these therapies include headaches, nausea, and sleep disorders.

CHAPTER FOUR

Exploring Options To Quitting Cold Turkey

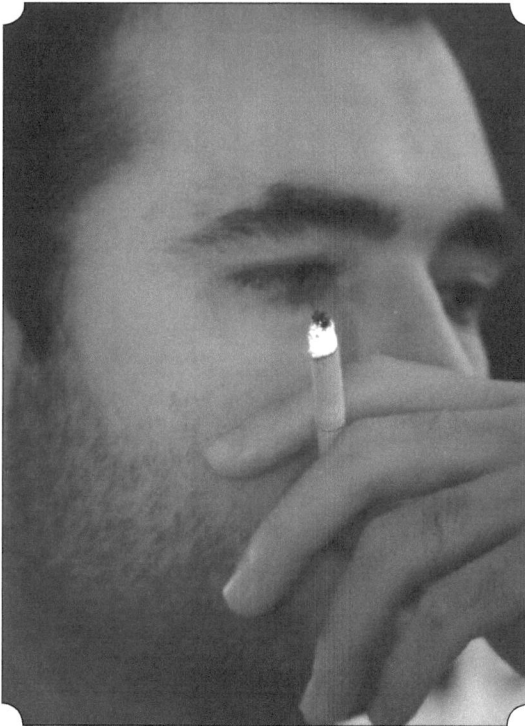

While quitting cold turkey is as popular a way to stop smoking as any, a growing number of smokers are exploring alternative therapies.

Nicotine addiction treatment centres around the world offer an array of different programs designed to ease the distress of withdrawal from nicotine.

Research is still being conducted on many of these individual therapies, but word of mouth recommendations clearly show they are effective for some smokers, and less so for others. If the reasons for smoking are as individual as the people who reach for cigarettes, so too are the methods for quitting.

Here are some other options for support when you quit smoking:

Hypnosis

Among the most popular of these alternative therapies are hypnosis, acupuncture, group help sessions and behavioural therapy. There is also a laser treatment designed to rid the body of nicotine and a Zyban Stop Smoking Treatment. Zyban is a kind of bupropion pill designed to help a person stop craving to have a cigarette in his mouth.

Hypnosis does have many disciples. What it does essentially is help the person who has just quit smoking to relax while they focus on a problem they are having and the desired result that they want. In hypnotherapy, the smoker relaxes completely, leaving his subconscious mind vulnerable to the planting of a suggestion.

In this case, the therapist plants the idea that the person is a non-smoker and the idea is that when the person comes out of hypnosis, his subconscious mind will accept that idea and help orchestrate the person's change of behaviour.

A host of studies have confirmed that hypnosis can be a very effective tool to quit smoking, with at least 66 percent of smokers finding success through it. It works because it reduces the smokers' stress and gives them techniques for controlling stress, and it prompts a change in attitudes and associations towards smoking.

Sometimes good results are recorded after only one visit. Some hypnotherapists prefer to offer multiple sessions to ensure success. Hypnosis can also be used with nicotine replacement therapies like the patch.

Acupuncture

Research shows that the people who seek out acupuncture treatments as an aid to stop smoking are extremely committed to making their quitting exercise a success.

While all clinics offering the treatment have some variations, the general format is that you will be asked to fill up questionnaires in advance that outline your smoking history, your health history, and your smoking triggers.

Proponents of acupuncture point out that it reduces the cravings and lessens the withdrawal symptoms associated with quitting. The sessions focus in particular on the first month of quitting, since this is usually the most difficult.

Usually four to five treatments are prescribed. Despite a popular theory that ear acupuncture works best for smokers, in reality the area treated is unique to each individual. Normally it is a combination of body puncture points with ear points.

The needles are inserted, and you will relax for about half an hour.

A review of the effectiveness of acupuncture treatments as aids to stop smoking was conducted by A.R. White, H. Rampes, and E. Ernst at the Department of Complementary Medicine, University of Exeter, UK. The researchers concluded that there is no clear evidence that acupuncture, acupressure, laser therapy or electrostimulation are effective for smoking cessation. That does not mean that they are not recommended; it just means that the verdict is still out. It still comes down to what works for you and all options should be considered.

Group Help And Behavioural Therapy

A number of people find it easier to withdraw from addictions through support groups or as individuals receiving private counselling. In many cases this is also combined with nicotine replacement therapy.

Sessions found to be the most effective were motivational interviewing and cognitive behavioural therapy.

Motivational Interviewing

In sessions of <u>motivational interviewing</u>, you will receive non-confrontational counselling intended to help you explore conflicts about changing your behaviour, identifying gaps between smoking and other life goals, and supporting the choice to quit.

For example, you may genuinely want to stop smoking, and you may assure your family of that. But privately, you are really worried that you will gain massive amounts of weight if you stop.

The idea behind motivational interviewing is to help you uncover conflicts like this and deal with them so they don't jeopardize your quitting process. The whole process is extremely non-judgmental.

Does it work? The science suggests that it does.

A recent study headed by Dr. Douglas Lai, a family medicine specialist in Hong Kong, showed encouraging results among more than 10,000 smokers who used motivational interviewing to quit between 1997 and 2008, compared to smokers who tried to quit after receiving just basic advice from a stop-smoking literature.

The interviewing program was most effective when delivered by the smoker's own doctor as opposed to another health care worker.

The findings were featured in The Cochrane Library, a publication of the Cochrane Collaboration, an international organization that evaluates medical research.

The idea of motivational interviewing as a method to help smokers was the brainchild of Dr. Stephen Rollnick and Dr. William R. Miller. They proposed that the counsellor in the motivational interview should elicit ambivalent feelings from the smoker, enabling him or her to have a free expression of all sides of the inner conflict. Without judging, the counsellors then help the smoker to find a resolution that includes a choice of a method to quit.

This technique has also been used to help people overcome asthma attacks, drug addiction, diabetes treatment problems and obesity.

If you decide to try motivational interviewing, you can expect the interview sessions to range from one 20-minute sessions to multiple sessions over several days, but the technique and strategy is always the same.

Cognitive Behavioural Therapy

In Cognitive Behavioural Therapy, a therapist will work with you on cognitive strategies to help you reduce your cravings.

For example, your might be encouraged to think about the health impact of smoking on those you love. This allows you to think about cigarettes in a different context, as something less pleasant than a relief from stress.

Does this work?

Again, the science supports it. Brain scans conducted on people engaged in cognitive behavioural therapy indicates that the therapy actually has a physical impact on the way the brain works, and that in turn, decreases the severity of the cravings the smokers endure.

The National Institute of Drug Abuse has expressed interest in this therapy as a means to helping other people overcome various addictions in the future.

The Institute funded the study on the use of Cognitive Behavioural Therapy with people who are trying to quit smoking and discovered how their brains were retrained with it. The therapy recipients experienced change in their prefrontal cortex, the place where we control our emotions. The therapy participants had a more active prefrontal cortex.

A second part of the brain, the striatum, which is related to our craving and reward-seeking behaviour, seems less active.

People who took the therapy also said their cravings were less intense.

Other Options

There are a host of alternative remedies offered to people trying to quit smoking and while many are harmless, few have been vetted by accepted scientific research published in peer reviewed journals.

Aromatherapy is considered an option for new quitters trying to make it through the early weeks.

Herbal remedies such as St. John's Wort and lobelia are touted by some as something to help the smoking in the stages of withdrawal.

Smokers Do Try Everything

One thing researchers have discovered about all the ways people seek help when they are trying to quit smoking is that the smoker who has tried and failed will often try again, but use a completely different support technique the next time.

But despite all the therapeutic options for help, an astoundingly large number of successful ex-smokers either quit cold turkey or quit by gradually decreasing the number of cigarettes they smoked.

CHAPTER FIVE

Create Your Personal Quitting Plan

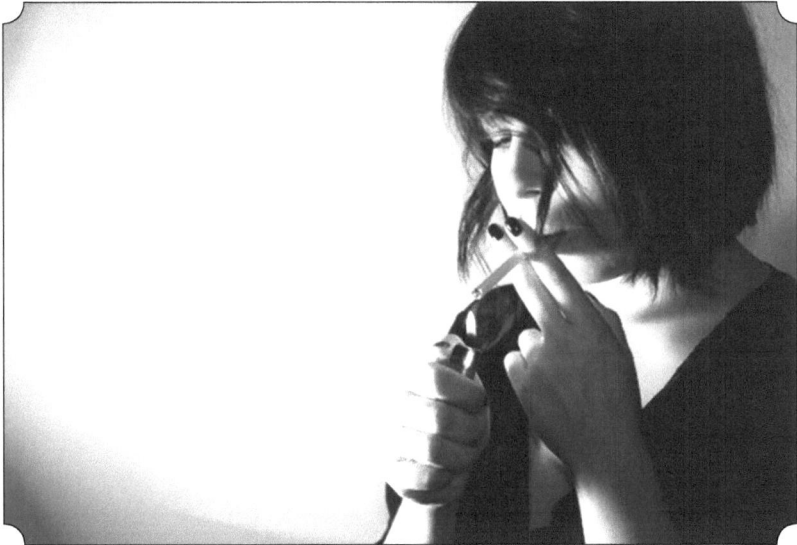

Quitting Smoking is one of the most important and difficult projects you will encounter in your life. So it makes sense to create a plan before you embark down this road, just as you would for any other significant endeavour.

The essence of your plan will be figuring out how you are going to deal with situations which are the triggers that now prompt you to reach for your cigarette, cigar or pipe.

If you have tried to quit before and failed, you need to first think about the strategies you tried and where they went off the rails. Knowing what didn't work is just as important as embarking on a strategy that you hope will work this time.

The first thing to do is to consult your calendar and pick a "quit date." It should be about two weeks away. If you are more inclined to smoke in your workplace than at home, pick a Saturday or Sunday to stop smoking.

If you smoke less during the week than on weekends at home, then start on a Tuesday when you are working. That way you will have a few days to build up your resolve before the weekend arrives.

Once you have set your date, your project now has edges. You begin to build.

How well your plan works will depend hugely on how well you know yourself and your smoking habits, so these next couple of weeks are crucial to rounding out your strategy. You are on a mission to study yourself.

You need to make time every day to think about a component of the plan, do your research about your habits, figure out your strategies, and get everything ready for your quit day.

Many smokers skip carelessly over this part, assuming that a few thoughts gathered in the back of their brains and a "rough idea" will suffice. While it's true that may work for some people, the truth is you have a much better chance of succeeding on this project if you actually write or type out your plan and keep it where it is accessible to you at all times.

Even if it is in a journal at home, type it up so you can send it to yourself as an email. You will need it when you least expect it.

Here is a draft of what your plan should consist of:

My Stop Smoking Plan

This is my reason to quit:

These are the top three situations in which I always reach for a smoke:

My main strategy to avoid smoking is:

This is the support technique I will use:

This is the quitting medication I will use:

My quit date is:

Now it's time to start filling in the details. In Chapter 1 you were encouraged to do some self-sleuthing and discover your main personal reason for wanting to quit. Non-smokers often assume that the decision to stop is always triggered by a realization that smoking is harmful to your health, but you know whether or not that's true.

You may have had a health scare and decided to take better care of yourself. You may be looking forward to the arrival of your first child and don't want to expose them to the health effects of second-hand smoke. Only you know your true motivation, so write it down and develop it.

If it is your child, paste a photo of your child's happy face next to "This is my reason to quit." Use your words to describe your reason along with a photo if that is possible. If you think you can save enough money for a vacation at a tropical resort by quitting, get a picture of your dream vacation spot and put it adjacent your "This is my reason to quit" step.

In the second step, write down the top three situations in which you consistently feel that you "must" have a smoke. Is it your Sunday night bridge club where all the guys or girls smoke like chimneys, the place where they will half-heartedly encourage you with words like "good for you, wish I could quit" and then go right on smoking in front of you?

Is it the shopping or sports trip you have planned next month where you share a room with your best friend, a life-long smoker who won't be quitting with you? Is it the minute you pick up a beer to savour in the neighbourhood pub? Is it after sex or after a nice meal? Is it mid-morning when you and a couple of co-workers step outside for a smoke break?

Pick three, just the top three, for these are the ones with the most potential to undermine your best endeavours. You will find that these triggers are usually tied to people, activities, events or places that you are seriously emotionally attached to, and that is why it will be tough to overcome them.

Many a smoker has been heard to say that when they quit smoking, they simultaneously quit their lives. So much of their social activities came wrapped up with the cigarette package, that they find themselves lost and ill at ease, unable to go to their old haunts or even visit the people whose company they enjoyed.

That is why in your master plan to quit smoking you have to figure out strategies to cope with your trigger situations.

You may develop a "quitting coach" or a "quitting buddy" who will resolve to talk you through the tough periods.

One way to get an idea if your strategies will work is to try them out in the two-week period leading up to your quit date. For example, you might decide that you could still step out for a break with your smoking work colleagues if you brought a cup of coffee with you, or a crossword puzzle to do.

You might find that you just can't endure the bridge game where everybody smokes, but you can start a new tradition with a couple of the people you really liked there, and instead go to the movies one night a week. When old behaviours don't work anymore, you need to think in advance of new behaviours that can replace them.

You might time your quit date with a period where you are going to be away on a course or a project for a month or two. You might begin as you go on your summer holiday, knowing that the stresses that make you reach for a smoke will be less as you are lying in the sun on the beach.

You might line up a big new project to preoccupy you so you don't miss the old habits as much. For example, you might find it easier to not drop by a bar and have a smoke with your friends if you decide to time your quitting with your urge to finally build the garage that you always wanted.

Pick one strategy and develop it. See how it adapts to most of the challenging social situations in which you will find yourself. Test it.

The next part of your plan is determining the kind of quitting medication you will use. In Chapter 2 and 4 we considered a number of options. You need to find the one that will work best for you, and again, if you can get a bit of practice time in with it before you quit, so much the better.

If you are addicted to nicotine, and you likely are if you have been smoking any amount of time, you will endure withdrawal symptoms when you quit. These symptoms look a lot like you being a grouch. You will be anxious and irritable and find it hard to focus. You may feel hungry all the time or not interested in eating at all.

Consider whether you are going to use nicotine patches, gums, inhalers or some other medication to help you go through the withdrawal symptoms.

Add your quit date to the plan, sign it, and you are ready to go.

Remember, from that date forward, you will not smoke, not even one cigarette. People who give in to the urge to "just have one" end up returning to their original smoking habits. There is no half-in, half-out approach to quitting.

In the coming chapters, we will take you through still more strategies to deal with the cravings, the stress and depression, the weight issues, and the accompanying life changes.

CHAPTER SIX

How To Deal With Cravings

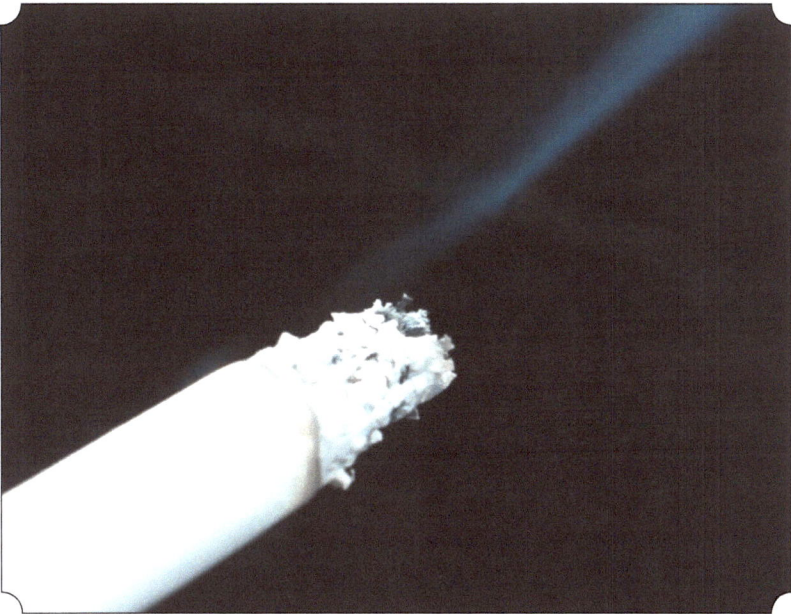

When you stop smoking, you can expect to endure about six gut-wrenching, mind-blowing, body-slamming craving episodes a day in the first week.

Slowly, in the second week, they will occur less often, dropping to about 1.4 cravings in 10 days.

Each episode lasts just under three minutes.

That means the moment you quit, you are setting yourself up each day for almost 20 minutes of being challenged to the core of your being.

What can you do to handle your cravings and save your sanity during this rough stage of your life?

You can use quitting products like nicotine patches and gums, you can change your environment so your normal triggers won't occur, you can use coping thoughts and techniques, and you can change your daily routines and habits to accommodate the new smoke-free you.

Quit coaches are unanimous that one of the most effective weapons in this mental war is substitution. If you used cigarettes as a reward, find something else to delight yourself. If you used cigarettes as comfort, find another source of feeling nurtured. If you used them to ease the stress in your life, try working on eliminating that stress through other avenues.

If you just smoked because you enjoyed it, the substitution theory is still valid. Just try to find some other function that you enjoy and that is less harmful to your health, and embrace it.

Even if you smoked in combination with something else you enjoy, like a cup of coffee or reading, find a substitute for that habit until you are strong enough to resume it.

For example, if you took a time out each morning for a cup of coffee and a cigarette before you jumped into the day's activities, try instead to drink a glass of fruit juice or a smoothie that first week. The dissociation from your normal routine will trick your brain and sooth the cravings, at least for awhile.

If you smoked after supper, try going for a walk instead or starting to play a new computer game.

When the craving catches you off guard, pull out your plan and remind yourself again of the number one reason why you quit.

If you and a friend or spouse quit at the same time, be a support system to each other. Many smokers find that by quitting on such big anti-smoking campaign days as Weedless Wednesday (in January in North America) or the World Health Organization's World No Tobacco Day May 31 each year, they immediately have a support system.

Why do such cravings accompany the cessation of smoking?

Because you have been feeding your body regular doses of nicotine through your cigarettes, your subconscious mind has developed nicotine use cues. At specific times, places, encounters with specific people, or waves of emotion, your subconscious cues kick in and expect a dose of nicotine. Your dopamine pathways send a message of "I want." This is when you feel a craving for a cigarette.

When you quit smoking, you begin a process of breaking and extinguishing smoking cues.

This is why when you stop smoking, you have to stick with the plan. If you relapse even once, you start the chain of chemical dependency again.

However, if you can be strong and get through the craving, they will fade. Your mind and body will be rid of all traces of nicotine within 72 hours. That is when the healing process starts and you begin to live your smoke-free life.

Within two to three weeks, you will have established the pattern of not smoking and will be strong enough to experience smoking triggers and find the power to resist them. However, science has yet to explain why years later certain social or emotional situations will still trigger a craving for a cigarette, even in a person who hasn't smoked for more than five years.

What is clear is that quitting is a lifestyle, not just a one-shot action.

As time passes, you can help cravings to come farther and farther apart by appreciating the value of your new lifestyle and confirming to yourself repeatedly that you are a non-smoker.

Forty Ways To Leave Your Cigarettes Behind

1. Change your reward system. Disengage yourself from the things that held you to your smoking habit. If you were happy, you rewarded yourself with a cigarette; if you needed a bit of comfort, you rewarded yourself with a cigarette. You now have to train your brain to accept a new reward system. Try putting a dollar in an envelope every time you get the craving and training your brain by imagining yourself having an enviable vacation.

2. Breathe deeply. Close your eyes, breathe deeply, and think about the real reason you are quitting. Give yourself a two-minute time out to think positively about your decision.

3. Consider it a life or death choice. Sounds tough, but think about giving into your craving in the same way you would think about stepping into the path of a speeding car. Is that step really worth dying for?

4. Chew gum. It takes the edge off the craving and keeps it at bay.

5. Fix what needs fixing. Think about your real reason for smoking. You may have reached for your cigarettes to relieve stress, give yourself a moment of quiet time, or escape boredom or unpleasantness. The problem is still there and needs fixing, cigarettes or no cigarettes. It's just more visible now that it's not view through a puff of smoke.

6. Understand that smoking did not make the times good. For many smokers, cigarettes are synonymous with the good times of life, the times out with friends, sex, and great meals. Think about how great they are all by themselves. You don't really need that cigarette to make them better.

7. Substitute habits for time spent with cigarettes. If you enjoyed a long and leisurely smoke every morning after the children left for school, find another way to savour a moment. Make your own espresso, whip up a smoothie. Create a substitute treat for yourself.

8. Drink water. Keep a big bottle of it handy. When you start to crave a cigarette, drink a glass of water instead. It will help greatly as you go through the nicotine withdrawal symptoms.

9. Suck on a tasty mint. Mint has a way of filling up your taste buds and the void that occurs when you stop smoking.

10. Keep busy. Start a creative new project that captures your imagination and tantalizes your mind. When cravings occur, focus on the new project.

11. Suck on long licorice sticks, carrot sticks or celery sticks.

12. Re-read your primary reason for quitting every time you get a craving.

13. Keep a journal. When the cravings hit, write about how you feel and when it ends, how good you feel about yourself. Writing helps reinforce our behaviour and validate it.

14. Talk to your friends and family about your decision to stop smoking. Tell them you may need their help to talk you through a craving. If they can support you for the first six months, tell them you will treat them to a great "smoke-free" barbecue.

15. Deliberately arrange your life around non-smokers. Of all your friends, invite the non-smoking couple to supper that first week. Go for a weekend away with your non-smoking friends.

16. If you are in a private situation or are in public but are a very accomplished singer, sing your way through a craving. Sing in the car, sing in the kitchen, and sing in the workshop. This has the double impact of activating your brain and your mouth and seems to reduce the cravings.

17. Keep your hands busy. Even if you are watching television or sitting talking on the telephone, doodle, take notes, draw cartoons, or anything that keeps you tied up.

18. Practice saying "no thanks, I don't smoke" in front of a mirror when you get a craving. Say it in a variety of tones and make a variety of faces. Reinforce to all aspects of your personality that you have stopped smoking.

19. Chew on straws or Popsicle sticks when you are watching television.

20. For the first month after you quit, plan one small reward for yourself every day that you endure.

21. Take walks on nature trails or city blocks where you will find interesting things to occupy your mind. You are less inclined to get a craving as you walk in the outdoors.

22. Take up a new hobby that occupies your hands, such as whittling or knitting.

23. Make your environment smoke free. Ask others not to smoke around you. Set up smoke-free zones in your car, in your home, and in your office. Book no-smoking rooms at hotels and no-smoking sections in restaurants to reinforce your smoke-free status and avoid temptation.

24. Reinforce your strategy to yourself. Tell yourself "I am happier not smoking," and "I don't want to smoke."

25. Fantasize about your rewards as a non-smoker. Think about breathing freely in your old age. Imagine running through fields of aromatic wildflowers.

26. Set short-term goals. Instead of saying you will never have another cigarette in your life, tell yourself you aren't going to smoke this morning, then this afternoon, then after supper and so on.

27. Rid yourself of all reminders of your smoking habit. Make sure all ashtrays are emptied, cleaned and stored away or given away.

28. Secure a supply of your nicotine replacement medication in advance of your quit date so that you do not run out at a crucial time early in the process.

29. Make sure your quit date comes at a time when you are relatively relaxed, not when you are under pressure to complete a huge project.

30. As you adapt to a new non-smoking routine, use it as the impetus to make other small changes in your daily routines. Walk a different trail, take a different route to work, or alter your normal nightly routines.

31. Drink water when you get a craving to smoke. Fill your mouth and let the water sit there for a few seconds. Swallow slowly, savouring the taste.

32. Reinforce what a good thing you are doing by using some of the money you save to reward yourself with a night at the movies or a concert or a meal out.

33. If you are feeling especially tense, this will be a high risk of reoccurrence day. Avoid temptation by going for a walk or working out at a gym or even reading a book of meditations or listening to calm music.

34. Keep a stash of a few favourite food treats you love in the drawers where you used to keep your cigarettes. When you reach for them out of habit, your mind will be distracted with the new idea of a tasty treat.

35. Take steps to control your social life. Instead of meeting friends in a bar where you expect most people will be smoking, invite a few friends over to a backyard barbecue or even a sit-down meal at your smoke-free home.

36. When you sit down to watch television, if that was a time you normally smoked, select a different chair instead. Look at the screen from a new perspective.

37. Take a shower as soon as you get up in the morning to replace a habit of reaching for your first cigarette of the day.

38. Brush your teeth as soon as you are done a good meal to discourage a craving for an after-dinner smoke.

39. Keep your fridge and shelves well stocked with healthy snacks. In the early days, a mid-morning cigarette break can be substituted with a short nutrition break.

40. Try to limit the amount of caffeine you drink. With the nicotine moving out of your system, your body will retain much more caffeine than previously.

CHAPTER 7

Strategies To Deal With Stress And Depression

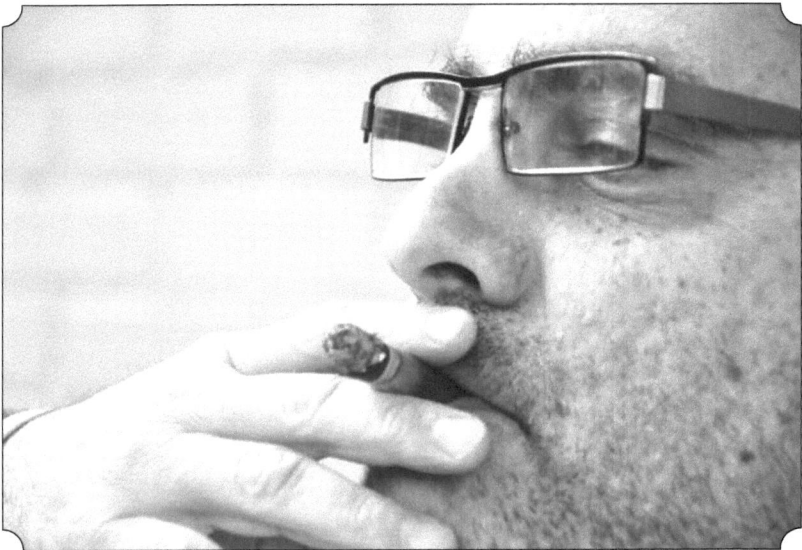

Monica smoked for 18 years. A long bout of pneumonia heightened her awareness of how it feels to have her breathing compromised, so she decided to quit for the fourth time.

She did great for five weeks. Then one evening she got into an argument with her husband and stormed out to get a package of cigarettes. She sat in her car and smoked half a pack, and by the next day, was right back to her pack a day habit.

Jim was driving a truck for long hours each day. When he quit smoking, he sailed through the first three weeks, singing along with the music on his radio, chewing gum, and staying tough.

One night, with waves of tiredness flooding over him and miles to go before settling into his own bed, he stopped at a gas station and lit up. He felt less lonely, less stressed, less tired, less put-upon.

Within a week, he felt addicted to nicotine again.

Stress, depression, anger and loneliness are the darker shadows hovering in the background when you decide to stop smoking. None of them appear strong enough to break your resolve alone, but taken in combinations of two and three, they can thwart your plans and destroy your quitting success.

When you are stressed, you will instinctively reach for comfort in whatever form works for you. When you are angry, you often bottle up your feelings to avoid conflict, and instead reach for a cigarette to set your world straight again. Loneliness will push a person to reach for a cigarette to fill up the minutes with what feels like a calming activity.

In our frantically scheduled world, fatigue is one of the worst enemies of quitting success. Being tired makes all the other negative emotions worse. Our stress is magnified, our loneliness more acute, and our anger more intense.

There is really only one effective strategy for handling the stress associated with quitting smoking. That is to totally adjust our thinking about the relationship between smoking and tension.

Right now you likely think that one of the reasons you enjoyed smoking so much is that it helped you relieve your stress and tension. Your body and your mind both tell you that is the truth. You know when you feel tense and you reach for a cigarette, within seconds you are experiencing a feeling of calm. As you slowly inhale and exhale, you think: "awww...this is great. This is what I am really going to miss about smoking.... this tension easing."

Now it is time to adjust your thinking.

How do you feel about the tension-relieving qualities of cigarettes when you discover that rather than helping you relieve stress, the nicotine in cigarettes was actually causing it? A number of scientific studies link smoking with psychological distress. Smokers also report a decreased satisfaction with life compared to non-smokers.

When you stop smoking, your negative feelings about life do not necessarily change. In fact, sometimes they get worse. In even the most positive people, smoking is often associated with negative mood changes. These negative moods heighten the incidents of craving cigarettes and are responsible for nearly half of smokers relapsing to their old life.

It is normal when you stop smoking to feel a degree of anxiety and depression as well as irritability. You may also have difficulty concentrating and be restless. It is reasonable to expect it may take up to three months for these symptoms to decrease.

By adapting strategies to deal with stress during the quitting process, you will come to look forward to a world where you find yourself calm in a crisis, no longer fuelled to a frenzy by the presence of nicotine in your body. You will experience a significant lack of anxiety within a few weeks, once your body adjusts to the changes.

Smokers who see cigarettes as a means of releasing their stress find it the hardest to get started on the quitting process. They keep putting it off on the grounds that things are tough right now and they don't want to make it worse by losing their tension-reducing tool

Research tells us there is no perfect time to quit. What is known is that the more times you decide to quit and then renege, the more tension you will experience on the subject.

Go into your quitting plan knowing and accepting that nicotine is a strong and powerful force, but that you are stronger. Arm yourself with treatments and techniques to wrestle its control away from you.

Know that you are most vulnerable to the impact of stress during the quitting process if your normal habit was to reach for a cigarette when you felt anxious. You need to recognize this and have an arsenal of other strategies to help you cope with those stressful moments.

It helps a great deal if you can change your mindset and instead of thinking about cigarettes as something you are taking away from your life, you think instead of all the benefits you are gaining with your action. This is a plus, not a minus, on the scale of life experiences.

You have to believe that you are capable of quitting. That self-knowledge and self-belief is essential if you are going to prevent yourself from sliding into a relapse.

Be aware that if you have a history of depression and you stop smoking, you may experience depressive symptoms or actual depression. This is a side effect of quitting. If you have a history of a mental health issue, you should take care to monitor your moods for any early signs that your condition is getting worse.

Talk to your family doctor before you quit smoking and early in the process if you experience worrisome symptoms. Be particularly aware of not isolating yourself from those who care about you.

Your family doctor may suggest exercises in mood management combined with therapy and counselling. When such help is offered, be sure to accept it. You will need support on your side of the nicotine battle.

A growing number of doctors are also experimenting with the prescribing of antidepressant medication. While there is a growing field of support for this trend, the verdict is still out on whether or not this is an essential intervention. Keep your confidence in your doctor and discuss what pharmacotherapy, if any, will be most effective for you.

It is important to manage the stress associated with quitting effectively before it impacts your physical well-being as well. Heightened tension and anxiety can boost your heart rate. It also can affect your breathing and cause muscle tensions. These physical changes in turn create more tension, starting a difficult and unproductive cycle.

Stress Buster Ideas For
The Early Weeks of Quitting

Change Your Routine

Get up an hour earlier in the morning and go for a walk in the fresh air. Give up an hour of television at night and instead go for a workout at your neighbourhood gym. Take up jogging or Nordic Walking. Sit in a different chair at your kitchen table for meals. All of these subtle changes of routine will help ease the discomfort of breaking a long-held routine of smoking.

Engage In New Eating Habits

Stock up on fresh fruit and vegetables, especially things like carrot and celery sticks that can be used to stave off cravings. You have taken a big step to enhance your health; why not go the rest of the way and move towards a healthier diet?

Banish Stress With Exercise

Start with the simple act of increasing your natural movements. Add 10 minutes to your daily gardening routine or park the car a block away from your workplace. Once you have incorporated these gentle changes into your routine, rev up your exercise plan with new programs like walking, running, and weight training.

Anecdotal evidence supports joining a team sport as you quit smoking. Many ex-smokers report the positive benefits of a supportive team and the joy of learning new skills in a fun atmosphere. This new focus helps to banish the stress of quitting.

Keep A Journal

A number of studies have shown that people who keep daily journals find them an effective way to decrease stress in their lives.

It is as if the act of putting thoughts into words, and then the exercise of writing them into a journal is cathartic. Journal-writers report their regular writing sessions, either daily or at least three times a week, help them to stay focused and organized in the process of making major life changes.

Keep The Rewards Coming

Modifying our behaviour is easier when we introduce a reward system, according to a number of scientific studies. When you quit smoking, include in your personal plan options for rewards to help you keep on track.

Make small rewards after each smoke-free week, and work together larger rewards after each smoke-free month. After six months invest in something you have always wanted to do, whether it is an indulgent full day or weekend at a spa or a camping trip and hike with a group of your best buddies. When the stresses of quitting threaten to undermine you, think about this upcoming experience and let it fill your focus.

Change What You Are Drinking

Both caffeine and alcohol can create stress when you quit smoking. Once the nicotine is removed from your body, the effects of caffeine are heightened and you may find having a couple of cups of coffee or cola drinks leaves you edgy and irritable.

By reducing or simply eliminating alcohol for a short time, you can avoid becoming extra nervous and cranky.

Practice relaxation techniques

Sit comfortably with your eyes closed and breathe deeply. Pay attention to the thoughts and feelings swirling around in your mind. Now focus on the things you can hear, the feeling of your body on the floor or mat, and slowly breathe in and out for about three minutes.

As you inhale and exhale, be conscious of the air coming in and out of your body.

Remind yourself of the cleansing process your body is enjoying, and the long-term benefits of this road you are travelling.

Reach Out For Help

If you know that you are likely to be vulnerable to stress during your quitting process, talk to your doctor in advance. Obtain a referral to a psychologist or professional quitting coach in your area.

Consider options like hypnosis or a program of meditation.

Take up yoga or some form of breathing or muscle relaxation exercises.

Create Your Own Meditation Exercise

If you have flexibility in your surroundings, build up your own three-minute meditation exercise. You need to have three minutes alone to make this effective, since that is the average time a craving attack will last.

Lie down or sit comfortably in a reclining chair. Close your eyes and breathe deeply. You will feel a rush of thoughts all pushing for priority in your mind. Let them bounce around each other.

Instead of dealing with any of them, turn your attention to the sounds you hear. Slowly let your awareness centre on the places where your body is touching the chair, the bed, or the floor.

Feel which parts of your physical body seem tense, and slowly and consciously try to relax them.

Pay attention now to your breathing. Concentrate on the relief of the air travelling into your lungs. Feel your body relax as you breathe out.

Repeat this cycle of being aware of closing your eyes, listening to the sounds, feeling your physical body tension, and breathing slowly in and out in a cycle for three minutes.

Do this each time you feel a craving or a bout of stress.

Get Enough Sleep

If you don't get sufficient sleep (seven to nine hours a night) when you stop smoking, you will be more prone to relapse. Studies show not only does sleep deprivation decrease your self-control, but it also diminishes your normal attention span and makes you feel extremely fatigue.

When you are in such a weekend state, it is easy to succumb to the temptation of a cigarette.

CHAPTER EIGHT

How To Keep The Weight Off During The Quitting Process

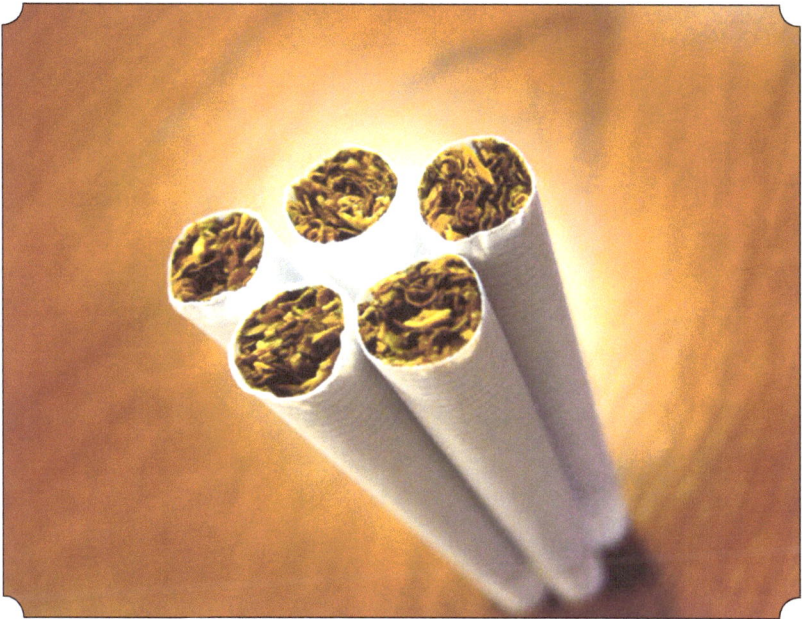

One of the factors that may keep you smoking long after you entertain the idea of quitting is the fear that you will gain a great deal of weight as soon as you stop.

55

You likely know some ex-smokers who successfully kicked the habit but are now moving around with an extra 20 pounds on their frame. You imagine yourself smoke-free, but afraid to look in the mirror and see that all of your favourite clothes are now too tight to look good on you.

There is some evidence that this is a realistic concern.

A 1991 student found that the average weight gain caused by people quitting cigarettes is 6.2 pounds (2.8 kg) for men and 8.4 pounds (3.8 kg) for women.

This is not a deal breaker in its own right. In fact, the researchers at the time concluded that weight gain is not likely to negate the health benefits of quitting, but its "cosmetic effects" may interfere with attempts to quit.

There is a reason why you may experience a small weight gain, even if you are extremely cautious with your diet. One study showed that a heavy smoker burned 200 more calories per day than a non-smoker, even when both were eating identical diets. Scientists suggest the reason for this might be nicotine's ability to increase energy metabolism. Another possible reason being studied is nicotine's effect on your peripheral neurons.

In 2012, The Cochrane Review, which reviews scientific studies, looked at another reason. There were claims made in a 2008 study that you could delay weight gain after quitting by using sustained-release bupropion, nicotine gum, and nicotine lozenges. They concluded, however, that there is still not sufficient data to confirm that link.

Overall, if you incorporate more exercise into your life as you quit smoking, and eat a healthy diet, you can maintain control of your weight as well as become more physically fit.

What you should not do is to start rewarding yourself with sweets, cakes, and other high-sugar foods as a reward for each day you don't smoke. When this happens, you are basically using food as a substitute for nicotine, and you are setting yourself up for another kind of unhealthy habit.

What can you do to avoid gaining weight when you stop smoking?

You may consider a behavioural intervention, also called behaviour therapy or management therapy. In this therapy, you will be counselled to try to change behaviours that would cause you to gain weight.

Your goal in this therapy, and in general as a successful life strategy, is to balance your energy intake with your energy output.

You can accomplish this either by reducing your food intake or increasing your physical activities, or combining programs to accomplish both aims.

Many smokers find when they first quit that they need to avoid caffeine or they will be irritable and sleepless. If this is happening to you, it is not your imagination.

When you stop ingesting nicotine into your body, your body responds by retaining more caffeine. This substance is in coffee and tea as well as cola drinks and chocolate. Too much caffeine leaves you restless and sleepless.

Keep in mind that when you stop smoking, your body retains more caffeine. This makes you even more restless and sleepless and more inclined to eat more than you should, especially sugar-laden snacks for a jolt of energy.

Try to understand what is happening in your body. The reason you are hungry focuses on your brain's dopamine, its primary motivation transmitter. If you are hungry, that is because your dopamine pathway from the brain is being stimulated. You may try to ignore it, but before long it becomes a persistent craving.

Instead of satisfying your cravings with fatty or sugary foods, try to substitute fresh fruit juice, flavoured water, or caffeine-free teas for the high-caffeine content drinks that were previously part of your diet.

Follow a well-balanced diet, with lots of fresh fruits and vegetables. Try to eat at regular times and not skip meals. Balance your day with low-fat snacks such as fruits and vegetables to keep fatigue at bay.

Don't skip a meal during the first few weeks after quitting. Going for a long time without eating has a tendency to cause your blood sugar levels to go down rapidly, and this can hinder your recovery.

This can be frustrating if you were able to skip the occasional meal when you were a smoker. You may wonder why your body has changed so much.

The point is that when you were smoking, you were constantly inhaling a dose of the stimulant nicotine. It gave you a quick kick because it was able to pump stored sugars and fats into your blood stream.

So even when you skipped a meal or even two, you usually were okay because you kept getting your regular doses of nicotine. That is why so many smokers insist that they keep smoking to stay slim.

But if you skip meals without the nicotine, the result is not at all what you hoped. Instead, you will be engulfed in feelings of nervousness and trembling, irritability and anxiety, and even anger and frustration.

Worse still, you may find it impossible to concentrate.

Instead eat three regular meals and at least two healthy snacks each day as part of your quitting plan.

Here are some eating strategies to keep your energy vital and eliminate the risk of giving up your stop-smoking campaign because you feel restless and fatigued:

Cut down on the "bad" things. Get the alcohol, cakes, cookies, chips and soft drinks right out of your house and your office drawers or mini-fridge. Rid yourself of temptation by ensuring you are not within easy reach of cookies, cakes, chips and soft drinks.

1. Cut down on alcohol.

2. Trim the visible fat from your meat.

3. Stash the fryer and instead cook on a grill or steam your food.

4. Decrease your use of butter, margarine, dressings, sauces and gravies.

5. Allow yourself a maximum of five snacks a day: one between breakfast and lunch in the morning, two between lunch and dinner in the afternoon, and one after dinner in the evening.

6. Don't let quitting smoking become your excuse to just indulge in whatever food you want. Instead make wise food choices and stick to a healthy eating plan. Monitor your weight regularly during the quitting process.

7. Remember that over the long term, your body after you quit smoking will likely look better than it did when you were smoking. Because smokers have a higher body fatness overall and an abnormal fat distribution from non-smokers, you will find in time after quitting that you will end up with a more ideal body shape than you had while smoking.

CHAPTER 9

Steps For Dealing With Stressful Social Situations

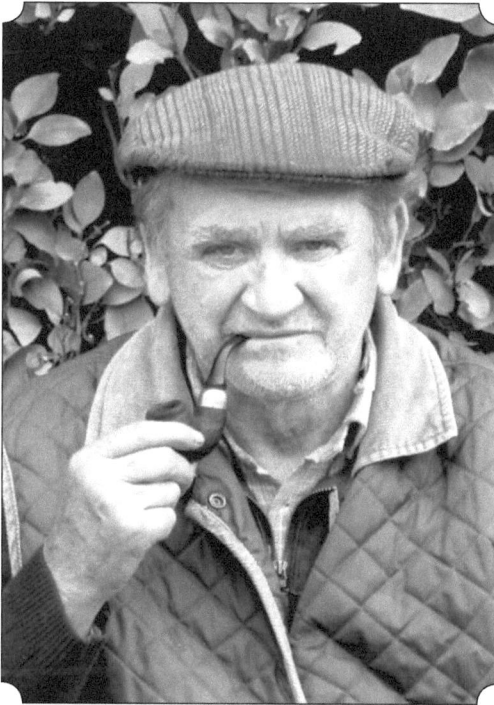

You will miss smoking when you are alone in the calmness and comfort of your own routines.

But you will miss it even more in social situations.

There is a huge social component to smoking, from slipping out for mid-morning smoke breaks with colleagues where support and shared stories bolster your spirits to having a few beers with your best friends on a Friday night.

In fact, some smokers actually describe themselves as "social smokers" just as there are "social drinkers." They rarely reach for their pack of cigarettes or a cigar when they are home alone, but put them in an environment where everyone is doing it, and they can't resist.

There is actually a class of smoker scientists have identified as a "chipper," a person who can chip in and smoke with the crowd and then never smoke again unless they find themselves in that same situation. This is not the norm.

Most people who start as "chippers" turn into full-blown nicotine addicts. They enjoy the way they feel in the social situation, and before long, they want to try to accomplish the same result at home.

People most inclined to smoke in social situations are also the ones who are most apt to relapse even after an absence of smoking for five, 10 or 20 years. They are in a mood of fellowship and friendship, and they assume, perhaps on the urging of others they care about, that they could have "just one." Sadly, they cannot.

A 2011 study of smokers who had been free of nicotine for even 30 years found that they still succumbed to their old smoking habits if they even agreed to just smoke one cigarette.

"Nearly all smokers who lapse experience a full-blown relapse," the researchers concluded.

Smokers who are strong enough to return to social settings where they once smoked and where others are still smoking have mixed responses. Some find it too painful to stay and realize that this is a part of their life they just have to give up if they are going to regain their smoke-free lifestyle.

But about half of smokers who have successfully quit report that they find it much easier than they thought to re-insert themselves into a social setting that they used to enjoy as a smoker. Those who are able to do that have managed to conquer the power of nicotine over them and no longer feel threatened in its presence.

Still another category reports being able to return to the social setting and resist smoking, but only if they don't drink either. It is a fact that cravings often appear strongest when you are having a drink in a social situation. It is likely in such instances that alcohol weakens your resolve.

The first time you feel ready to go back into a social situation in which you previously smoked and where you will likely encounter friends who are still smoking, make sure you have a planned strategy before you step in the door.

Practice saying "no thanks, I don't smoke" in front of the mirror until you look and feel comfortable saying it.

Have an escape plan in place. Tell your friends you can only stay for a few minutes because you have to pick up your spouse or child somewhere, but that you just wanted to see them.

If the time of your alleged appointment arrives, you might want to leave and make sure that your first social encounter is a good one.

Repeat the same strategy the next time. If your allotted time to leave arrives and you still feel strong, you can also call the person you were supposed to pick up (having arranged the charade in advance) and discover that you don't have to leave for another half hour. Keep allowing yourself timed escape valves until you know you are strong enough to stay for an entire event without relapsing.

Find substitutes in social situations to replace what smoking used to mean to you. For example, if it was your habit to leave the chatter of a cocktail party and step outside for a few minutes to enjoy the quiet, and you used a cigarette to accomplish that, try to find another reason.

Step outside to make a phone call to a person who is supporting you. Visit the washroom and spend a minute or two away from the crowd to collect your thoughts and your resolve. Go outside to look at a car, a garden, a landscape. Plan your reason in advance, even if you are the only person you need to convince.

Think about all the reasons you normally reached for a cigarette in a social situation. Was it to calm yourself or collect your thoughts, to avoid boredom, to get away from the lull of the chatter?

Now think about alternate ways to accomplish the same things. Armed with your new strategies, try them out. When they work well, keep them in your behaviour arsenal to ensure that you do not lapse. If you try a strategy and still feel stressed and close to losing control, make a quick exit and think about why it didn't work, and what might work better the next time.

Here are the top 10 tips successful quitters used to gently get themselves back into the social world where they once smoked:

1. Take a baby step before leaping into your old environment. Suggest going to a movie where nobody is allowed to smoke, for example, so you can see your friends who still smoke but not feel compelled to join them.

2. Spend time calmly promising yourself that you will not smoke on the social occasion in which you plan to participate. After all, successful quitting is just meeting one challenge at a time.

3. Try to take a quitting buddy or non-smoking friend with you for essential support if you need it. If they see you close to lapsing back with a promise of "just one," they should pull out your number one reason for quitting. Nobody really has to say another word.

4. Don't drink in situations where you normally drank and smoked together for several weeks until you build up your resolve.

5. When you are ready to have a drink, hold it in the opposite hand from where you usually held it, in other words, in the hand where you would normally hold your cigarette. This sends a subtle message to your brain that you have changed.

6. Keep your hands and mouth busy. Nibble on an appetizer. Sip water or an alcoholic beverage. Check your emails on your mobile phone. Chew gum.

7. Say "no thanks, I don't smoke" instead of just "no thanks" when someone offers you a cigarette. It creates an end to the situation. If you say "no thanks, not just now" you leave yourself open to be tempted again later.

8. If you feel insecure about how to behave because you are not smoking, just observe what people who aren't smoking are doing.

9. Remember that there is nothing wrong and no big explanation needed if you feel yourself in danger of losing control and you just want to go home. Get up and go. People will understand.

10. Don't be lulled into a false sense of security that you can have "just one" cigarette and then leave them alone again.

CHAPTER 10

Build On The New You: Find New Habits To Replace Old Ones

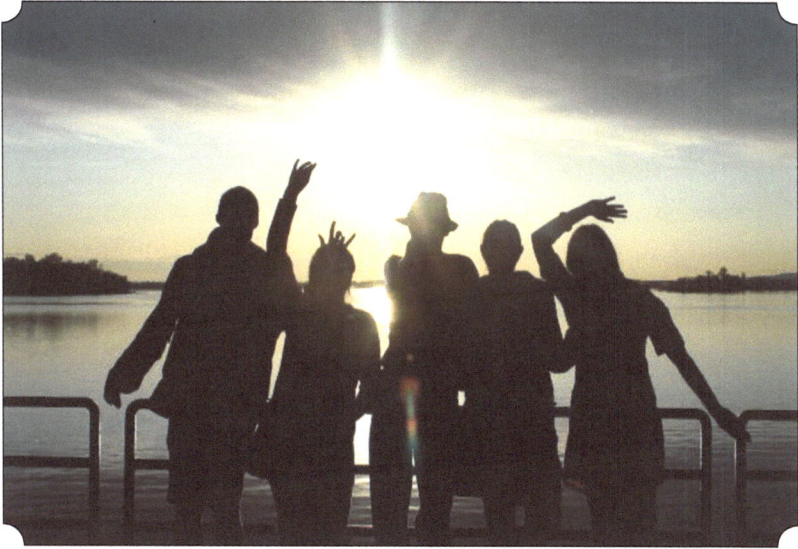

Quitting smoking is one of the biggest and most significant lifestyle changes you can make.

You have given up something you used to enjoy for a whole variety of good reasons and you are gaining in confidence each day.

But how do you fill that void?

The first thing to remember is that unlike television's imaginary characters, real people don't usually manage to completely change their life on a whim and stick with it. We need time to process the change, to get comfortable with it, and to practice it over and over again until it becomes part of the new us.

Being kind to yourself and taking new steps only as you feel ready is the foundation for your success. When it gets right down to it, the decision to quit smoking and find a way to stay smoke-free for life is highly individualized. You can be inspired or assisted by others, but you ultimately have to go your own way if your new habit is to become part of who you are.

The only consideration is that you should ensure that in filling the void that not smoking has creating, you don't rush to replace one addiction with another. If you substitute food for smoking, your health will suffer. If you substitute gambling for smoking, you will ultimately be unhappy all over again.

Instead, use the weeks after you get past the cravings to consider what you really want out of life and create a plan to achieve it. You may want to use the money saved from your smoking habit to travel and see the world. You may want to go back to school or university and try to find a more challenging career.

Do not be in a great hurry to fill up the void. A little emptiness is like a blank slate. It is a place where creativity can flourish and where something better than what we started with can be developed.

Try to continue journaling for as long as possible. Write your thoughts not just about smoking, but about other things you observe from your new smoke-free vision. Think about your motivations for change, and what else they might prompt you to do.

When you decided to quit smoking, you made up an individual plan to sustain you through the tough times. The number one task was determining why you really wanted to quit smoking.

Why not use this second phase of your life create a second individual plan? Knowing you can do one of the hardest things in the world, the next challenge should be a lot easier.

Figure out your motivation for another change in life. Figure out a strategy to accomplish it. Make your plans and go for it!

Warning Signs You Are In Trouble

For the rest of your life, you have to remember that you are susceptible to nicotine addiction, and you must remain vigilant.

Here are three signs that you are in danger of relapsing:

1. You are taking puffs off somebody else's cigarette. - Don't fool yourself. You are very, very close to buying your own. Ask your friends and family to show their love and support for you by refusing you if you ask for a puff of their cigarette or even a cigarette. Make it clear you want them to be firm, no matter how much you cajole.

2. You start to rationalize that you could return to smoking on a limited program. – If you start to think

that if you could just smoke on Poker Night or Ladies' Night Out, just once a month, stop that thinking immediately. You can't make it work. Nobody can.

3. You question whether being tough for so long is really worth the effort. – It is. You can and will get through this. Treat yourself to something else you really enjoy.

What To Do If You Relapse

Do not let one cigarette derail your efforts to quit. It can happen. You have a really bad craving and you give in. The worst possible thing you can do is throw up your hands, say "well, that's it, I've failed" and got buy a pack.

Instead, think about the length of time that you were able to quit. Remind yourself of how strong and accomplished you felt to manage that. Realize that you have slipped up only once.

Resolve to get back on track. No excuses! Remember that you aren't the first smoker and you won't be the last to try and fail before you succeed for good.

Think about the circumstances that caused you to fall off your plan and consider how to avoid them in the future..

Most of all, remember the reason you quit in the first place.

www.ingramcontent.com/pod-product-compliance
Lightning Source LLC
Chambersburg PA
CBHW051235090426

42740CB00001B/29